The Vegan Diet

50 Quick & Tasty Recipes to Eat Healthy Food and living the Vegan Lifestyle

Naomi Fields

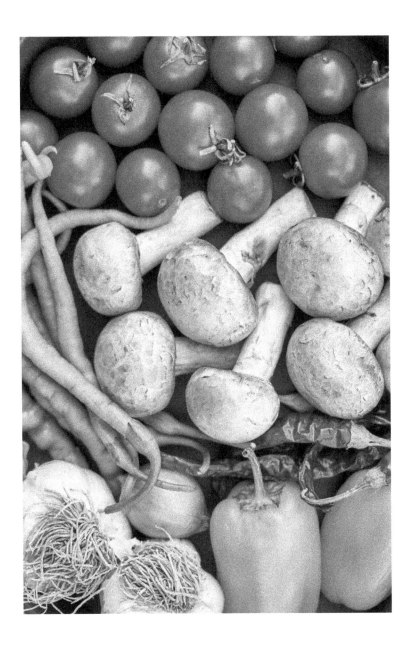

Table of Contents

Introduction

Plants (such as vegetables, grains, nuts, and fruits) and plant-based foods make up a vegan diet.

Vegans avoid foods derived from plants, such as dairy products and eggs.

As a vegan, you should eat healthily.

A diverse and healthy vegan diet can provide you with the majority of the nutrients you need.

For a vegan diet that is both safe and delicious:

1. Per day, consume at least 5 portions of a variety of fruits and vegetables.
2. Potatoes, bread, rice, pasta, or other starchy carbohydrates may be used as a foundation for meals (choose wholegrain where possible)
3. Dairy substitutes, such as soya drinks and yoghurts, are available (choose lower-fat and lower-sugar options)
4. consume some beans, pulses, and other protein-rich foods
5. Select unsaturated oils and spreads, and eat in moderation.
6. drink a lot of water (the government recommends 6 to 8 cups or glasses a day)

If you choose to include high-fat, high-salt, or high-sugar foods and beverages in your diet, do so in moderation.

Vegan sources of calcium and vitamin D

Calcium is needed for strong bones and teeth.

Dairy foods (milk, cheese, and yoghurt) provide the majority of calcium for non-vegans, but vegans may get it from a variety of sources.

Calcium-rich foods for vegans include:

1. spinach fortified unsweetened soya, rice, and oat drinks green, leafy vegetables – such as broccoli, cabbage, and okra, but not spinach fortified unsweetened soya, rice, and oat drinks
2. Tofu calcium-set
3. pulses of sesame seeds and tahini
4. bread (both brown and white) (in the UK, calcium is added to white and brown flour by law)
5. Raisins, prunes, figs, and dried apricots are examples of dried fruit.
6. To minimize the effect of sugar on teeth, a 30g portion of dried fruit counts as one of your five a day, but it should be consumed at mealtimes rather than as a snack between meals.

Vitamin D is needed by the body to control calcium and phosphate levels. These nutrients support the health of your bones, teeth, and muscles.

Vegans can get vitamin D from the following sources:

- sunlight exposure, particularly late March/early April to the end of September – Before your skin begins to turn red or burn, remember to cover it up or shield it (see vitamin D and sunlight)
- unsweetened soya beverages, fortified fat spreads, and breakfast cereals (with vitamin D added)
- supplementing with vitamin D

- Check the label to make sure the vitamin D in a food isn't from animals.

Iron sources for vegans

The formation of red blood cells requires iron.

While iron from plant-based foods is absorbed less well by the body than iron from meat, a vegan diet may be high in iron.

Iron-rich foods for vegans include:

- dark green, leafy vegetables such as watercress, broccoli, and spring greens wholemeal bread and flour breakfast cereals fortified with iron
- apricots, prunes, and figs are examples of dried fruits.

Vitamin B12 vegan sources

Vitamin B12 is needed by the body in order to maintain healthy blood and a healthy nervous system.

Vitamin B12 is commonly obtained from animal sources such as poultry, fish, and dairy products. Vegans may need a vitamin B12 supplement due to a lack of available sources.

Vegans can get vitamin B12 from the following sources:

1. unsweetened soya beverages fortified with vitamin B12 yeast extract, such as Marmite, which is fortified with vitamin B12 Vegan sources of omega-3 fatty acids
2. When consumed as part of a balanced diet, omega-3 fatty acids, such as those found in oily fish, can help maintain a healthy heart and reduce the risk of heart disease.

Vegans can get omega-3 fatty acids from the following sources:

- Oil from Flaxseed (Linseed)
- Rapeseed Oil
- Soybean Oil and Soy-Based Foods Like Tofu Walnuts

Plant Sources of Omega-3 Fatty Acids Do Not Have the Same Benefits in Lowering The Risk Of Heart Disease As Those Found In Oily Fish, According To Research.

If you eat a vegan diet, you can also take care of your heart by consuming at least 5 servings of a variety of fruits and vegetables every day, avoiding foods high in saturated fat, and keeping track of how much salt you consume.

Chapter 1: Breakfast recipes

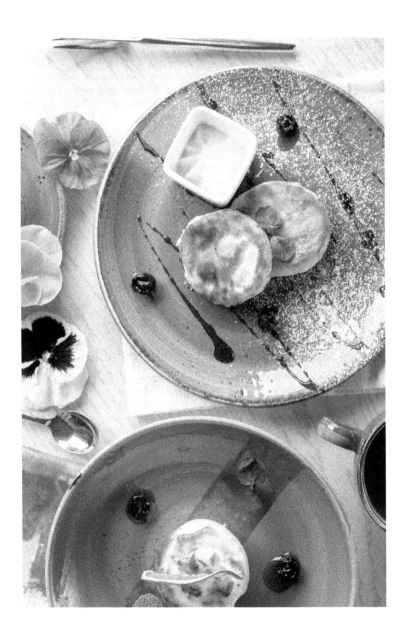

1. BUCKWHEAT PORRIDGE

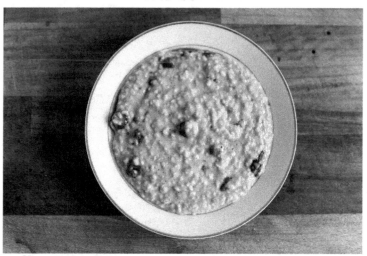

Ingredients
- 165 g buckwheat groats
- 750 ml unsweetened Almond Milk
- 1 cinnamon stick
- 1 teaspoon alcohol-and gluten-free pure vanilla extract generous pinch of sea salt
- 4 tablespoons maple syrup 150 g mixed berries
- 2 tablespoons unsweetened shredded coconut, toasted

Directions
1. Put the buckwheat groats in a saucepan and add the almond milk, cinnamon, vanilla and salt. Cover and cook over a medium heat, stirring occasionally, until the buckwheat is tender and has absorbed the milk, about 20 minutes. Discard the cinnamon stick.
2. Divide the porridge between 4 bowls.
3. Drizzle each portion with 1 tablespoon of the maple syrup, top equally with the berries, and sprinkle with the toasted coconut. Serve.

Nutritional Facts: 340 kcal; 70gr Carbs; 12gr Protein; 3gr Fat.

2. SPROUTED BUCKWHEAT MUESLI

Ingredients

- 330 g buckwheat groats 100 g raw pecans
- 50 g raw walnuts
- 20 g raw pumpkin seeds
- 20 g shelled raw sunflower seeds 80 gun sweetened shredded coconut
- 2 crisp, tart apples, grated down to the cores 2 teaspoons ground cinnamon
- 1 litre unsweetened Nut Milk
- 4 tablespoons maple syrup (optional)

Directions

1. Put the buckwheat groats in a bowl and cover with 1 litre filtered water. Set aside to soak for 2 hours at room temperature.
2. Drain the buckwheat in a colander and rinse well. Transfer to a shallow container, cover with a clean tea towel and leave to sit at room temperature until the groats begin to sprout, at least 8 hours or even overnight. Rinse and drain well.
3. While the buckwheat soaks, combine all the nuts and seeds in a bowl. Cover with about 5 cm of filtered water and set aside to soak at room temperature for 2 to 4 hours. Drain and rinse.
4. Put the sprouted buckwheat in a large bowl, add the soaked nuts and seeds, the coconut, grated apples and cinnamon and stir to combine.
5. Divide the muesli between 4 serving bowls and pour in 250 ml of the nut milk. Drizzle 1 tablespoon maple syrup, if using, over each portion and serve.

Nutritional Facts: 320 kcal; 50gr Carbs; 9gr Protein; 5gr Fat.

3. ROASTED NUTS AND SEEDS

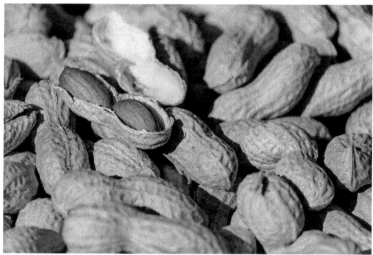

Ingredients
1. 1 cup raw sunflower seeds (or dry roasted without salt)
2. 1 cup raw pumpkin seeds
3. 2 cup raw almonds
4. 1 cup raw walnut pieces or halves
5. 1 cup raw pecan pieces or halves
6. 1 cup raw peanuts (or dry roasted without salt)
7. 1 cup raw cashew pieces or halves
8. 3/4 cup raw hazelnuts
9. 1/2 cup pistachios, roasted and salted

Directions
- Roast nuts separately by type in single layer on cookie sheets lined with parchment paper or foil. Roast at 350 degrees for the following times:
- Almonds - 20 minutes
- Walnuts, pecans, hazelnuts - 15 minutes
- Cashews, peanuts - 10 minutes
- Sunflower and pumpkin - 5-7 minutes (can be added without roasting if you like)
- Pistachio nuts - I have only found them roasted and salted, so they are the only added salt in this recipe.

Warning - when the nuts are fresh out of the oven, the aroma is so tempting, it might draw the family into the kitchen. Stand by with wooden spoon in hand to protect your recipe from marrauders!

- After the nuts cool, I package 1/4 cup serving in zip-lock snack bag, then store the bags in a gallon freezer bag. They will stay fresh for weeks, or they freeze beautifully

Nutritional Facts: 150 kcal; 12gr Carbs; 4gr Protein; 9gr Fat.

4. VEGGIE OMELET

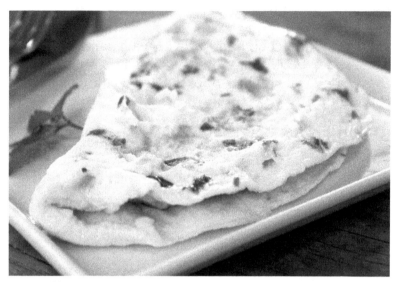

Ingredients

* 1/4 cup onion, chopped
* 1/4 cup green bell pepper, chopped
* 1/4 cup mushrooms, chopped
* 5 egg whites
* 1 whole egg
* 1 tablespoon skim milk
* 1/4 teaspoon salt
* 1/8 teaspoon ground black pepper
* 2 tablespoons Swiss cheese, shredded

Directions

* Coat a medium-sized nonstick skillet in cooking spray and place over medium heat. Add the onions, bell peppers, and mushrooms and cook for 3-4 minutes, or until tender.
* Meanwhile, in a small mixing bowl, add the eggs, milk, salt, and pepper. Beat until well combined.
* Remove the vegetables from the skillet and set aside. Re-coat the skillet in cooking spray and add the egg mixture. Cook for 2 minutes or until the bottom of the eggs begins to set. Using a spatula, gently lift the edges of the egg

and tilt the pan so the uncooked egg flows toward the edges.
- Continue to cook for 2 – 3 minutes or until the center of the omelet begins to look dry. Add the cheese and vegetables to the center of the omelet. Using a spatula, fold the omelet in half. Cook for another 1 – 2 minutes, or until cheese is melted and egg has reached desired consistency.

Nutritional Facts: 170 kcal; 10gr Carbs; 10gr Protein; 10gr Fat.

5. POWER-UP MILLET BREAKFAST BOWL

Ingredients

1. 2 tablespoons (30 ml) avocado oil, divided
2. 2 cups (140 g) sliced mushrooms
3. 2 cups (298 g) cherry tomatoes
4. Sea salt and black pepper to taste
5. 1 cup (200 g) millet, cooked according to the package directions
6. 4 cups (80 g) arugula
7. 4 large pastured eggs, cooked to your liking
8. ¼ cup (38 g) goat cheese crumbles

Directions

- In a large skillet over medium heat, heat 1 tablespoon (15 ml) of the avocado oil. Add the mushrooms and tomatoes. Sauté for 5 to 7 minutes until the tomatoes burst and the mushrooms have started to brown. Set aside.
- Drizzle the remaining 1 tablespoon (15 ml) of avocado oil into the hot millet, then season it with salt and pepper to taste. Evenly divide the millet among 4 bowls.
- Top each bowl with one-fourth of the sautéed mushrooms and tomatoes, 1 cup (20 g) of arugula, and 1 egg. Sprinkle each with 1 tablespoon (about 9 g) of goat cheese.

Nutritional Facts: 250 kcal; 18gr Carbs; 18gr Protein; 13gr Fat.

6. QUINOA POWER MUFFINS

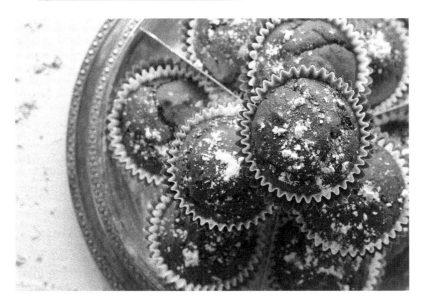

Ingredients

- 1 1/2 cups all purpose flour
- 2 teaspoons baking powder
- 1/2 teaspoon baking soda
- 2 packets stevia or other natural sweetener
- 2 teaspoons cinnamon
- 1/2 teaspoon salt
- 3/4 cup wheat bran
- 1/4 cup oat bran
- 3 tablespoons ground flax seed
- 1 1/3 cups almond milk
- 1/3 cup canola oil
- 1 teaspoon vanilla extract
- 1 cup quinoa, cooked
- 1/2 cup walnuts, chopped
- 1/2 cup vegan chocolate chips
- 1/2 cup hemp seeds

Directions

- Preheat oven to 400°F. Coat a 12-cup muffin pan in cooking spray.
- In a large mixing bowl, add the flour, baking powder, baking soda, stevia, cinnamon, and salt. Whisk together, then pour in the wheat bran, oat bran, and flax seed and whisk until thoroughly combined.
- In a separate bowl, add the almond milk, canola oil, and vanilla extract. Whisk together, then pour in the quinoa and whisk to combine. Pour the dry ingredients in and mix together with a wooden or plastic spoon. Fold in the walnuts, chocolate chips, and hemp seeds. Be careful not to overmix, there should still be some chunks.
- Pour the batter into the muffin pan, only filling each cup to 3/4 full. Place in oven and bake for 20 – 22 minutes, or until a toothpick inserted into the middle comes out clean.

Nutritional Facts: 150 kcal; 30gr Carbs; 5gr Protein; 3gr Fat.

7. PEANUT BUTTER & PROTEIN PANCAKES

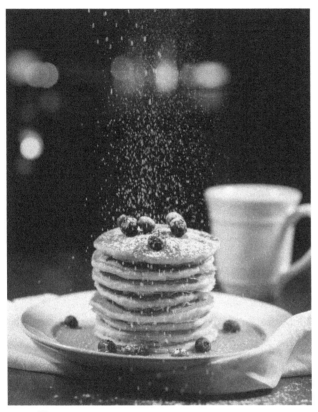

Ingredients

- 1/2 banana, mashed
- 2 teaspoons peanut butter
- 1 serving protein powder (of your choice)
- 1/3 cup whole grain pancake batter
- 1 teaspoon honey

Directions

- In a large mixing bowl, add the banana, peanut butter, protein powder, and batter and mix well.
- Coat a large nonstick skillet in cooking spray and place over medium heat. Divide the batter evenly in half and

spoon onto the skillet. Cook, turning when tops are covered with bubbles and edges look cooked. Drizzle honey on top.

Nutritional Facts: 100 kcal; 10gr Carbs; 3gr Protein; 5gr Fat.

8. AVOCADO LATKE "TOAST"

Ingredients

Yam Latkes

- 3 cups grated Japanese white yam (or any type of yam/sweet potato)
- ¾ cup grated white onion
- 1 small jalapeño, seeds and ribs removed, finely chopped (optional)
- ¼ cup plus 2 tablespoons ground flaxseed
- ½ teaspoon garlic powder
- ½ teaspoon black pepper
- ¼ cup avocado oil
- 3 pasture-raised egg whites, beaten

Fennel Slaw

- 1 large fennel bulb with fronds
- 10 fresh mint leaves, torn
- 2 tablespoons sundried tomatoes, chopped
- 1 small shallot, finely chopped
- 2 tablespoons fresh lemon juice
- 1 tablespoon extra virgin olive oil
- 1⁄8 teaspoon sea salt
- ¼ teaspoon black pepper

Smashed Avocado

- 1 large avocado, halved and pitted
- ½ cup fresh cilantro, tightly packed
- Juice and zest of 1 lime
- 1 small jalapeño, seeds and ribs removed, finely chopped (optional)
- 1 tablespoon extra virgin olive oil
- ¼ teaspoon black pepper

Soft-Boiled Eggs

- 4 pasture-raised eggs

Directions

- Preheat the oven to 375°F and line a baking sheet with parchment paper.
- For the latkes: Add the grated yams and onion to a fine strainer and press to remove excess moisture. In a large bowl, mix the jalapeño (if using), ground flaxseed, garlic powder, pepper, avocado oil, and egg whites together. Add the yams and onions and mix well until combined.
- Pack the mixture into a ¼-cup measuring cup and turn out each latke onto the sheet. Use your hands to flatten. You should have 8 latkes minimum. Bake for 15 minutes, flip, and bake for another 15 minutes until golden brown and crispy.
- Prepare the salad by removing the stalks and fronds from the fennel bulb. Coarsely chop the fronds and thinly slice the stalks. Place in a large bowl. Using a mandoline, thinly slice the bulb, cutting it in half if necessary. Add the fennel to the bowl along with the torn mint and chopped sundried tomatoes.
- In a separate small bowl, add the minced shallots, lemon juice, olive oil, salt, and pepper.
- Prepare the smashed avocado by scooping the avocado into a small bowl and roughly mashing it. Add the cilantro, lime juice, lime zest, jalapeño (if using), olive oil, and pepper. Mix until combined but chunky.
- To make the soft-boiled eggs, bring a large saucepan of water to a boil over medium-high heat. Using a slotted spoon, carefully lower the eggs into the water one at a time. Cook for exactly 6½ minutes, adjusting the heat to maintain a gentle boil. Transfer the eggs to a bowl of ice water and chill for 2 minutes. Once cooled, gently crack the eggs and peel.
- Combine the fennel mixture with the dressing. Assemble the dish by layering one yam latke with smashed avocado, adding another latke, then a scoop of salad, and topping with an egg. Repeat to make 4 total and serve.

Nutritional Facts: 154 kcal; 36gr Carbs; 14gr Protein; 8gr Fat.

9. PROTEIN OATCAKES

Ingredients

- 1/2 cup old-fashioned oats
- 1/2 cup fat-free cottage cheese
- 6 egg whites
- 1/2 teaspoon cinnamon
- 1/2 teaspoon vanilla extract
- 1/8 teaspoon baking powder
- 1 scoop vanilla whey protein powder

Directions

- Place all ingredients in a large mixing bowl and mix with a whisk or electric hand mixer until it thickens into a batter.
- Coat a large nonstick skillet in cooking spray and wipe away the excess with a paper towel. Save this for wiping the pan after cooking each pancake. Heat the skillet over medium heat.
- Pour or ladle about 1/2 cup of the batter onto the skillet and cook, 2 – 3 minutes each side until golden brown. Repeat for remaining batter.

Nutritional Facts: 45 kcal; 6gr Carbs; 1gr Protein; 2gr Fat.

10.   SPINACH AND TOFU SCRAMBLE

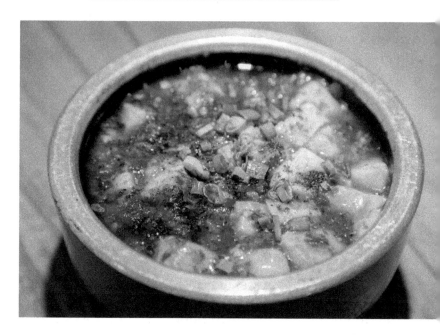

Ingredients

- 2 tomatoes, diced
- 2 cloves garlic, minced
- 3/4 cup fresh mushrooms, sliced
- 1 cup spinach, rinsed
- 2 1/2 cups firm or extra firm tofu, crumbled
- 1/2 teaspoon low-sodium soy sauce
- 1 teaspoon lemon juice
- salt and ground black pepper, to taste

Directions

- Coat a medium-sized skillet in cooking spray and place over medium heat.
- Add the tomatoes, garlic, and mushrooms and sauté for 2 – 3 minutes.
- Reduce heat to medium-low and add the spinach, tofu, soy sauce, and lemon juice. Cover with a tight fitting lid

and cook for 5 – 7 minutes, stirring occasionally. Sprinkle with salt and pepper.

Nutritional Facts: 230 kcal; 10gr Carbs; 25gr Protein; 10gr Fat.

11.   TEMPEH HASH

Ingredients
- 12 ounces tempeh, cut into 1/2-inch cubes
- 4 medium potatoes, peeled and diced
- 1 onion, diced
- 2 tablespoons low-sodium soy sauce
- 1/2 teaspoon garlic powder
- salt and ground black pepper, to taste

Directions
- Place the potatoes in a large pot, add water until the potatoes are just covered. Bring to a boil over medium-high heat and cook for 10 – 15 minutes, or until tender.
- Coat a large skillet in cooking spray and place over medium heat. Add the onions, potatoes, tempeh, and soy sauce and sauté. Stir frequently, ensuring you cook all sides of the tempeh cubes. Remove from heat and add the garlic powder, salt, and pepper.

Nutritional Facts: 250 kcal; 30gr Carbs; 10gr Protein; 10gr Fat.

Chapter 2 : Super Power Smoothies

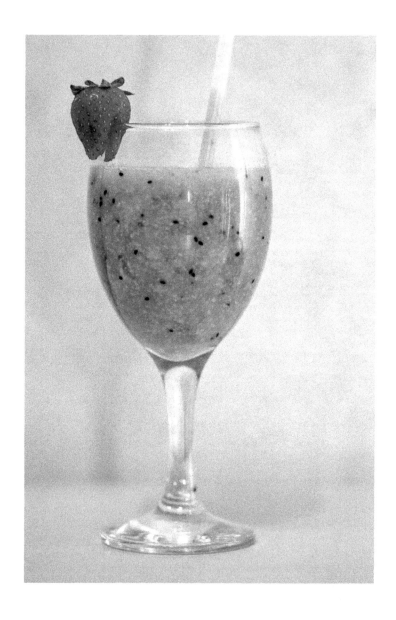

12. COCONUT-ACAI SMOOTHIE

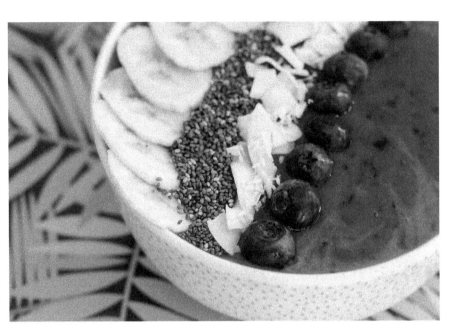

Ingredients
- 90 g frozen acai, cut into small chunks
- 2 tablespoons chopped raw shelled pistachios 1 date, pitted
- 2 teaspoons fresh lemon juice 300 ml Coconut Milk
- ½ teaspoon vanilla powder

Directions
1. Combine all the ingredients in a blender and blend on high speed until smooth and creamy, about 45 seconds. Drink immediately.

Nutritional Facts: 420 kcal; 67gr Carbs; 9gr Protein; 12gr Fat.

13.   MANGO-COCONUT SMOOTHIE

Ingredients
2. 165 g frozen mango chunks
3. 375 ml coconut water (or unsweetened nut milk or filtered water)
4. 2 tablespoons hemp seeds
5. 2 tablespoons coconut butter

Directions
- Combine all the ingredients in a blender and blend on high speed until smooth and creamy, about 45 seconds. Drink immediately.

Nutritional Facts: 80 kcal; 13gr Carbs; 1gr Protein; 3gr Fat.

14.   CHERRY BOMB SMOOTHIE

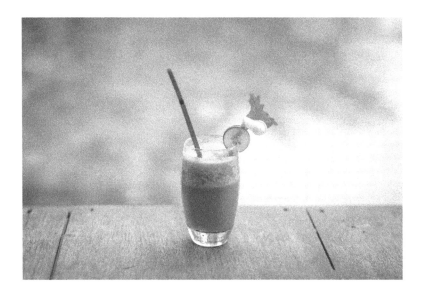

Ingredients
- 375 ml unsweetened Hazelnut Milk
- 120 g frozen pitted sweet cherries
- ½ teaspoon ground cinnamon
- ½ teaspoon freshly grated nutmeg
- ½ teaspoon ground ginger
- ½ teaspoon alcohol-and gluten-free pure vanilla extract (or ¼ teaspoon unsweetened vanilla powder)
- 1 tablespoon coconut butter

Directions
1. Combine all the ingredients in a blender and blend on high speed until smooth and creamy, about 45 seconds. Drink immediately.

Nutritional Facts: 70 kcal; 17gr Carbs; 2gr Protein; 0gr Fat.

15.   BANANA-RASPBERRY-COCONUT SMOOTHIE

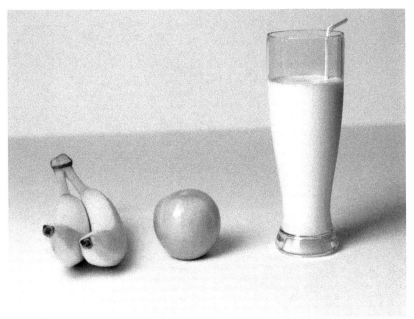

Ingredients
- 250 ml coconut water (or filtered water), chilled 1 banana, peeled and frozen
- 120 g frozen raspberries
- 2 tablespoons coconut butter 1 tablespoon coconut oil
- 60 g baby spinach

Directions
1. Combine all the ingredients in a blender and blend on high speed until smooth and creamy, about 45 seconds. Drink immediately.

Nutritional Facts: 250 kcal; 45gr Carbs; 11gr Protein; 4gr Fat.

Chapter 3 : Entrèe Recipes

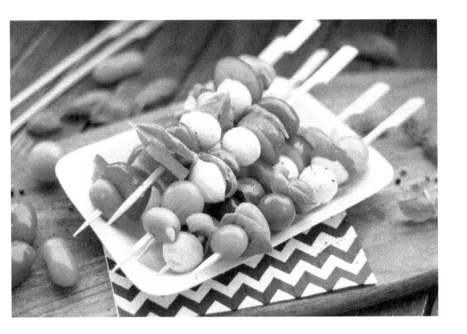

16.   TEMPEH TACOS WITH AVOCADO-LIME CREAM SAUCE

Ingredients

- 1 (6 ounce) block tempeh, cubed
- 1 teaspoon extra-virgin olive oil
- 1 teaspoon low- sodium soy sauce
- 1 teaspoon maple syrup
- 1/4 teaspoon ground black pepper
- 1 teaspoon vegan Worcestershire sauce
- 1/2 teaspoon barbecue seasoning
- 1/4 teaspoon cumin
- 1/8 cup cashews, soaked in water overnight
- 1/2 small avocado
- 2 tablespoons lime juice
- 1/4 cup water
- 1/2 teaspoon seasoned salt
- 4 (6 inch) corn tortillas
- 4 tablespoons salsa

Directions

- In a large ziplock bag, combine the tempeh, olive oil, soy sauce, maple syrup, pepper, Worcestershire sauce, barbecue seasoning, and cumin. Seal and toss, place in refrigerator for at least 2 hours or overnight.
- Heat a large skillet over medium-high heat and coat in cooking spray. Add the tempeh and sauté for a couple minutes, until browned and crispy.
- Meanwhile, drain the cashews. In a blender or food processor, add the cashews, avocado, lime juice, water, and seasoned salt. Blend until smooth.
- Top tortillas with equal portions of the tempeh and desired amount of lime sauce and salsa.

Nutritional Facts: 380 kcal; 40gr Carbs; 15gr Protein; 15gr Fat.

17.   TOFU PUTTANESCA

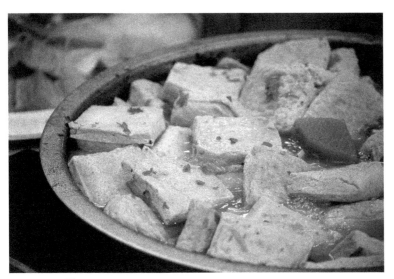

Ingredients

- 1 pound extra firm tofu, cubed
- 4 cloves garlic, thinly sliced
- 1/2 teaspoon crushed red pepper flakes
- 4 roma tomatoes, diced
- 2 tablespoons fresh thyme, chopped
- 2 tablespoons fresh oregano, chopped
- 1/2 cup mixed olives, chopped
- 1 tablespoon capers
- salt and ground black pepper, to taste

Directions

- Coat a large skillet in cooking spray and place over medium heat. Once hot, add the garlic and sauté for 1 – 2 minutes, until lightly browned.
- Add the tofu and red pepper flakes and sauté for about 10 minutes, or until tofu is browned. Add another coat of cooking spray after a couple minutes to prevent burning.
- Add the tomatoes, thyme, and oregano and cook for about 5 minutes, or until tomatoes have broken down.

Add the olives, capers, salt, and pepper and sauté for another minute or until flavors have mixed.

Nutritional Facts: 300 kcal; 50gr Carbs; 10gr Protein; 5gr Fat.

18.   BLACK BEAN BURGERS

Ingredients
- 1 can (15 ounce) black beans
- 1/2 onion, diced
- 1 teaspoon garlic powder
- 1 teaspoon onion powder
- 1/2 teaspoon seasoned salt
- 1/2 cup whole grain flour
- 2 slices whole grain bread, crumbled

Directions
- Coat a large skillet in cooking spray and place over medium heat. Add the onions and sauté until soft, about 3 – 5 minutes.
- Meanwhile, in a large mixing bowl, add the black beans and mash until only a few chunks remain. Add the onions, garlic powder, onion powder, salt, and whole grain bread. Add the flour in slowly, a couple tablespoons at a time, to prevent clumping.
- Divide into 3 portions and form into patties. Re-coat the skillet you used for onions in cooking spray and fry the patties until slightly firm, 2 – 3 minutes on each side.

Nutritional Facts: 100 kcal; 20gr Carbs; 5gr Protein; 1gr Fat.

19.   QUICK BEAN & SQUASH STEW

Ingredients

- 1 1/2 cups onion, chopped
- 1 1/2 cups green bell pepper, chopped
- 2 teaspoons minced garlic
- 1 tablespoon whole grain flour
- 2 cups butternut squash, peeled and cubed
- 2 (16 ounce) cans low-sodium diced tomatoes, with liquid
- 1 (15 ounce) can red kidney beans, drained and rinsed
- 1 (13 ounce) can baby lima beans, drained and rinsed
- salt and ground black pepper, to taste

Directions

- Coat a large saucepan in cooking spray and place over medium heat.
- Add the onion, bell pepper, and garlic and sauté until tender, about 7 minutes. Stir in the flour and cook for 1 minute.
- 3. Add the remaining ingredients and bring to a boil. Reduce heat and simmer 10 –   15 minutes, or until beans are tender.

Nutritional Facts: 200 kcal; 30gr Carbs; 10gr Protein; 3gr Fat.

20.   RAW ALMOND FLAXSEED BURGERS

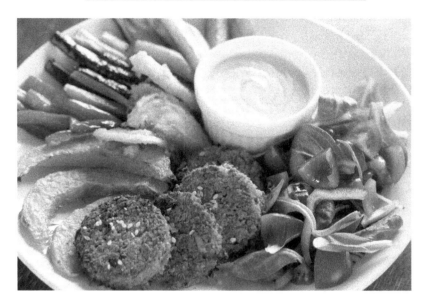

Ingredients

- 1 clove garlic
- 1 cup raw almonds
- 1/2 cup ground flaxseed
- 2 tablespoons balsamic vinegar
- 1 tablespoon coconut oil
- 1/4 teaspoon salt

Directions

- Place all ingredients in a food processor or blender and blend until well combined.
- Remove from food processor. Divide mixture evenly and shape into four patties.

Nutritional Facts: 100 kcal; 5gr Carbs; 10gr Protein; 10gr Fat.

21.   SQUASH & TOFU CURRY

Ingredients

- 2 tablespoons curry powder
- 1/2 teaspoon salt
- 1/4 teaspoon ground black pepper
- 1 pound low-fat extra-firm tofu, cubed
- 1 large delicata squash, halved, seeded and cut into 1-inch cubes
- 1 medium onion, chopped
- 2 teaspoons fresh ginger, grated
- 1 (14 ounce) can "lite" coconut milk
- 1 teaspoon brown sugar
- 8 cups kale, chopped and stems removed
- 1 tablespoon lime juice

Directions

- In a small mixing bowl, add the curry powder, salt, and pepper.
- Combine to make seasoning. In a large mixing bowl, add the tofu and 1 teaspoon of the seasoning, toss to coat.
- Coat a large nonstick skillet in cooking spray and place over medium-high heat. Add the tofu and cook, rotating every 2 minutes, until browned, about 8 minutes total. Transfer to a plate and set aside.
- Recoat the skillet in cooking spray, add the squash, onion, ginger and the rest of the seasoning. Cook, stirring occasionally, until the vegetables are tender and lightly browned, about 5 minutes.
- Stir in the coconut milk and brown sugar, bring to a boil. Add half of the kale and cook until slightly wilted, about 1 minute. Add the remaining kale and cook for an additional minute.
- Place the tofu back in the pan and mix well. Cover and cook, stirring occasionally, until the squash is tender, about 4 – 5 minutes. Remove from heat and stir in lime juice.

Nutritional Facts: 250 kcal; 30gr Carbs; 15gr Protein; 15gr Fat.

Chapter 4 : Side Recipes

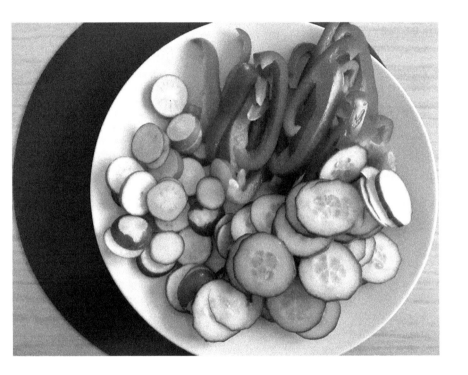

22.   SALTY EDAMAME

Ingredients
- 1 cup edamame, in the shell
- salt, to taste

Directions
1. Place a large saucepan over medium-low heat. Add 2 quarts water and edamame. Cover and let simmer until tender, about 5 – 8 minutes.
2. Drain and sprinkle with salt.

Nutritional Facts: 250 kcal; 6gr Carbs; 20gr Protein; 15gr Fat.

23.   THREE BEAN SALAD

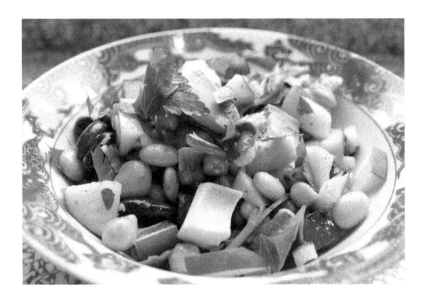

Ingredients

- 1 (16 ounce) can green beans, drained and rinsed
- 1 (16 ounce) can yellow wax beans, drained and rinsed
- 1 (16 ounce) can red kidney beans, drained and rinsed
- 4 tablespoons stevia or other natural sweetener
- 2/3 cup vinegar
- 1/4 cup vegetable oil
- 1/2 teaspoon salt
- 1/2 teaspoon ground black pepper
- 1 onion, sliced thinly

Directions

- In a large mixing bowl, add the stevia, vinegar, oil, salt, and pepper and whisk together to make the dressing. Pour in the beans and onions and toss to coat.

- Cover and place in refrigerator for at least 4 hours or overnight to chill, best if stirred occasionally. If desired, you can drain the excess liquid before serving.

Nutritional Facts: 150 kcal; 10gr Carbs; 3gr Protein; 10gr Fat.

24.   <u>EASY WHITE BEAN SALAD</u>

Ingredients

- 2 (15 ounce) cans Great Northern beans, drained and rinsed
- 1/2 pound plum tomatoes, chopped
- 1/2 cup fresh basil leaves, chopped
- 1 teaspoon salt
- 1/2 teaspoon ground black pepper
- 3 cloves garlic, minced
- 4 tablespoons extra-virgin olive oil

Directions

- Coat a large nonstick skillet in cooking spray and place over medium heat. Add the garlic and sauté until just lightly browned, 1 – 2 minutes.
- Meanwhile, in a large salad bowl, add the beans, tomatoes, basil, salt, and pepper. Pour the garlic and oil over the salad and toss to combine.
- Let the salad sit at least 30 minutes to allow flavors to combine.

Nutritional Facts: 200 kcal; 25gr Carbs; 10gr Protein; 10gr Fat.

25.   ITALIAN STYLE SNAP PEAS

Ingredients
- 1 large leek (white part only), washed, halved lengthwise and cut into 2-inch strips
- 1 pound sugar snap peas, trimmed
- 2 teaspoons extra-virgin olive oil
- 1/2 teaspoon salt
- 1 cup cherry tomatoes, halved
- 1 teaspoon dried oregano

Directions
- Preheat oven to 425°F. Coat a baking sheet in cooking spray.
- In a large mixing bowl, add the leeks, peas, olive oil, and salt. Toss to combine.
- Spread mixture out on baking sheet and roast for 15 minutes. Stir in the tomatoes and roast for 10 more minutes, or until vegetables start to brown. Sprinkle with oregano.

Nutritional Facts: 100 kcal; 8gr Carbs; 3gr Protein; 5gr Fat.

26.   CORN & EDAMAME SUCCOTASH

Ingredients

- 1 tablespoon canola oil
- 1/2 cup red bell pepper, chopped
- 1/4 cup onion, chopped
- 2 cloves garlic, minced
- 2 cups fresh corn kernels
- 3 tablespoons dry white wine
- 1 1/2 cups edamame beans, cooked according to package
- 2 tablespoons rice vinegar
- 2 tablespoons fresh parsley, chopped
- 2 tablespoons fresh basil, chopped
- 1/2 teaspoon salt
- 1/4 teaspoon ground black pepper

Directions

- Place a large nonstick skillet over medium heat, add the oil and heat. Once hot, add the bell pepper, onion, and garlic. Sauté until vegetables are tender, about 2 minutes.
- Stir in the corn, white wine, and edamame and continue to sauté for about 4 minutes, until flavors are well combined.
- Remove from heat and stir in the vinegar, parsley, basil, salt, and pepper.

Nutritional Facts: 100 kcal; 15gr Carbs; 6gr Protein; 5gr Fat.

27.   ASIAN GINGER BROCCOLI

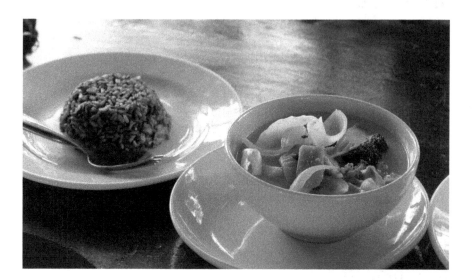

Ingredients

- 1 tablespoon canola oil
- 2 tablespoons minced garlic
- 4 teaspoons fresh ginger, minced
- 5 cups broccoli crowns, halved
- 3 tablespoons water
- 1 tablespoon rice vinegar

Directions

- Heat the oil in a large skillet over medium-high heat. Add the garlic and ginger and sauté until fragrant, about 45 seconds. Add the broccoli and sauté until broccoli is bright green, about 2 minutes.
- Pour in the water, stir and cover. Reduce heat to medium and cook until broccoli is tender, about 3 minutes. Toss with vinegar.

Nutritional Facts: 75 kcal; 5gr Carbs; 3gr Protein; 5gr Fat.

28.   SAUTÉED CAULIFLOWER

Ingredients

- 4 cups cauliflower florets, chopped
- 2 tablespoons water
- 2 teaspoons red wine vinegar
- 1 cup grape tomatoes, halved
- 2 tablespoons fresh parsley, chopped
- 1 tablespoon minced garlic
- 1/4 teaspoon salt
- 1/4 teaspoon ground black pepper

Directions

- Coat a large nonstick skillet in cooking spray and place over medium heat. Add the cauliflower, cover and cook for 4 minutes, stirring occasionally.
- Pour in the water and vinegar, stir to combine and cover. Let cook until cauliflower is golden and tender and the liquid has evaporated, about 4 more minutes.
- Add the tomatoes, parsley, garlic, salt, and pepper. Cook until tomatoes have softened and flavors have combined, about 2 more minutes.

Nutritional Facts: 120 kcal; 5gr Carbs; 20gr Protein; 10gr Fat.

29.   GASPACHO

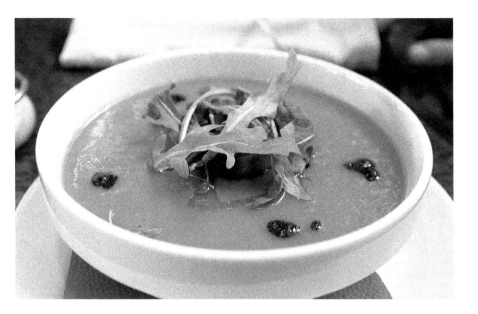

Ingredients
- 4 c. tomato juice
- 3 large ripe tomatoes
- 1 c. diced cucumber
- 1 c. chopped green bell pepper
- 1/2 c. chopped onion
- 1/4 c. red-wine vinegar
- 2 tbsp. olive oil
- 1 tbsp. minced garlic
- tsp. hot-pepper sauce
- chopped cilantro

Directions
- Put 2 cups of the tomato juice and half of the tomatoes, cucumber, bell pepper and onion into a blender or food processor. Add vinegar, oil, garlic and hot-pepper sauce. Process until almost smooth. Pour into a large bowl.

- Stir in remaining juice and vegetables. Cover and refrigerate at least 2 hours. Garnish with cilantro just before serving.

Nutritional Facts: 90 kcal; 6gr Carbs; 1gr Protein; 5gr Fat.

30.   GUACAMOLE

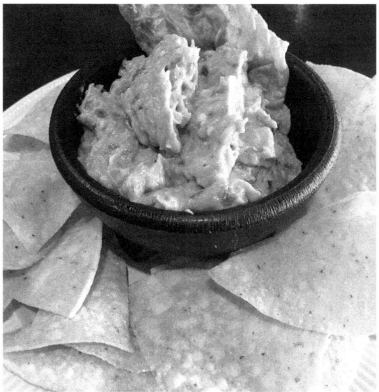

Ingredients
- 3 avocados - peeled, pitted, and mashed
- 1 lime, juiced
- 1 teaspoon salt
- ½ cup diced onion
- 3 tablespoons chopped fresh cilantro
- 2 roma (plum) tomatoes, diced
- 1 teaspoon minced garlic
- 1 pinch ground cayenne pepper (Optional)

Directions
- In a medium bowl, mash together the avocados, lime juice, and salt. Mix in onion, cilantro, tomatoes, and

garlic. Stir in cayenne pepper. Refrigerate 1 hour for best flavor, or serve immediately.

Nutritional Facts: 100 kcal; 5gr Carbs; 1gr Protein; 10gr Fat.

31.   HEARTY TOMATO SALAD

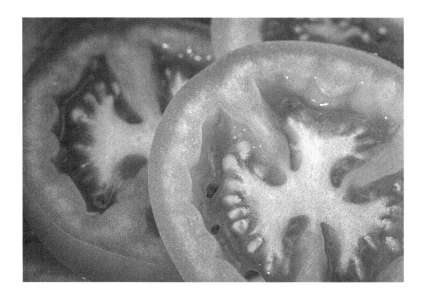

Ingredients
- 3 cups Cherry tomatoes, cut in half (works well with fresh, diced tomatoes too)
- 3 Garlic cloves, minced 1 tbsp
- 1 tbsp Olive oil
- 1 tbsp Balsamic vinegar
- 2 tbsp Lemon juice
- 4 Fresh basil leaves, julienned
- 1/2 tsp Salt
- 1/4 tsp Pepper

Method
- Mix all ingredients together in a medium sized bowl.
- Marinate for a minimum of 2 hours. Tomatoes can be stored in the refrigerator for up to 24 hours. For best results, bring to room temperature before serving.

- Serve over crusty bread, pasta, soft scrambled eggs or tossed into your favorite salad.

Nutritional Facts: 100 kcal; 25gr Carbs; 3gr Protein; 1gr Fat.

Chapter 5: Lunch Recipes

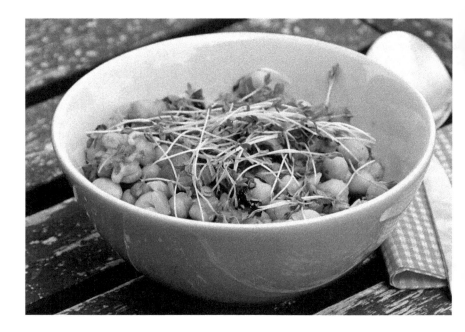

32.<u>SOUP</u>

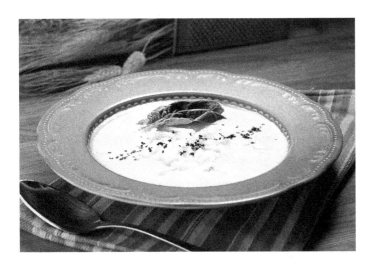

Ingredients
- 2 Tbsp water (or sub oil of choice // such as avocado or coconut)
- 2 cloves garlic minced (or sub 2 Tbsp garlic-infused oil*)
- 2 small shallots (optional // or 1/2 white onion as recipe is written // diced)
- 4 large carrots (thinly sliced)
- 4 stalks celery (thinly sliced)
- 1/4 tsp each sea salt and black pepper (divided // plus more to taste)
- 3 cups yellow or red baby potatoes (roughly chopped into bite-size pieces*)
- 4 cups vegetable broth (plus more as needed)
- 2-3 sprigs fresh rosemary or thyme (I used a bit of both)
- 1 cup uncooked green or brown lentils (thoroughly rinsed and drained)

- 2 cups chopped sturdy greens (such as kale or collard greens)

FOR SERVING optional
- Fresh parsley
- Brown Rice, White Rice, or Cauliflower Rice
- Garlic & Herb Flatbread
- Spelt Dinner Rolls

Instructions

- Heat a large pot over medium heat. Once hot, add water (or oil), garlic, shallots/onion (optional), carrots, and celery. Season with a bit of salt and pepper and stir.
- Sauté for 4-5 minutes or until slightly tender and golden brown. Be careful not to burn the garlic (turn heat down if it's cooking too quickly.)
- Add potatoes and season with a bit more salt and pepper. Stir and cook for 2 minutes more.
- Add vegetable broth and rosemary or thyme and increase heat to medium high. Bring to a rolling simmer. Then add lentils and stir. Once simmering again, reduce heat to low and simmer uncovered for 15-20 minutes or until lentils and potatoes are tender.
- Add your greens, stir, and cover. Cook for 3-4 minutes more to wilt. Then taste and adjust flavor as needed, adding more salt and pepper for overall flavor, vegetable broth if it's become too thick, or herbs for earthy flavor.
- Enjoy as is or serve with rice, cauliflower rice, or a side of flatbread or rolls (links above). I love garnishing mine with a little fresh parsley for a pop of color and freshness (optional).
- Store leftovers covered in the refrigerator up to 5 days or in the freezer up to 1 month. Reheat on the

stovetop and add more vegetable broth to rehydrate as needed.

Nutritional Facts: 150 kcal; 20gr Carbs; 15gr Protein; 10gr Fat.

33.   RISOTTO

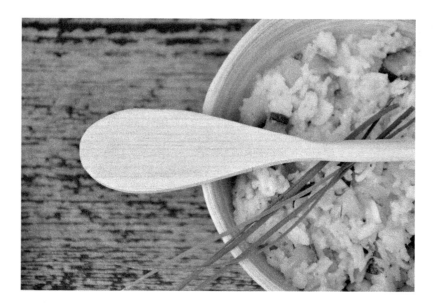

Ingredients
- 3 tbsp olive oil
- 1 large brown onion, finely chopped
- 2 medium carrots, cut into roughly 1cm/½in chunks
- 2 celery sticks, trimmed and cut into roughly 1cm/½in chunks
- 2 garlic cloves, finely chopped
- 275g/9¾oz risotto rice, such as Arborio
- 100ml/3½fl oz dry vermouth or white wine (optional)
- 1 litre/1¾ pint stock (made with 1 vegetable or chicken stock cube)
- 2 good pinches dried flaked chilies (crushed chillies)
- 1 small lemon, finely grated
- 50g/1¾oz Parmesan or vegetarian hard cheese, finely grated, plus extra to serve
- salt and freshly ground black pepper
- freshly chopped parsley, to serve (optional)

Method
- Heat the oil in a large saucepan or medium flameproof casserole. Add the onion, carrots and celery, stir well then cover and cook over a low heat for 10–12 minutes, or until soft and lightly browned, stirring 2–3 times to prevent it sticking. Add the garlic and cook for 2 minutes more, stirring.
- Stir in the rice and cook for a minute, stirring constantly. Pour in the vermouth (or wine, if using) and bring to a simmer. Cook for 30–40 seconds, stirring.
- Add all the stock and the chilli. Bring to a gentle simmer and cook uncovered for 22–25 minutes, or until the rice is tender and very creamy. Stir every 4–5 minutes for the first 10 minutes of the cooking time, then more regularly as the liquid reduces and the rice swells; stirring constantly for the final 5 minutes.
- Stir in the lemon zest and hard cheese. Season to taste with salt and pepper and serve topped with extra Parmesan and freshly chopped parsley if you like.

Nutritional Facts: 440 kcal; 70gr Carbs; 10gr Protein; 7gr Fat.

34. QUINOA SALAD

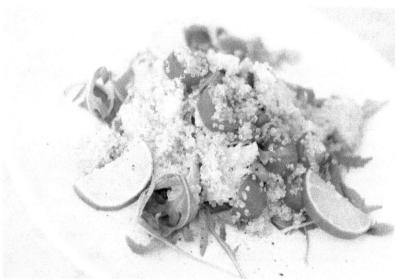

Ingredients
- 3 1/2 cups leftover cooked quinoa* (chilled)
- 1 large red bell pepper
- 2 cups diced English cucumber
- 1 1/2 cups grape tomatoes, halved
- 1 medium carrot, shredded (1/2 cup)
- 1/2 cup chopped red onion, rinsed under cold water in a sieve and drained
- 1 (14.5 oz) can chick peas, drained and rinsed

Dressing
- 1/3 cup olive oil
- 3 Tbsp fresh lemon juice
- 2 Tbsp red wine vinegar
- 1/3 cup chopped fresh parsley (chop somewhat fine)
- 1/4 cup chopped fresh cilantro (chop somewhat fine)
- 2 garlic cloves, minced (2 tsp)
- Salt, to taste

Directions

- Roast red pepper directly over the flame of a gas stove or under broiler, turning occasionally using metal tongs, until charred all over. Transfer to a container and cover and let rest 10 minutes, then peel**, core and seed and chop pepper.
- Meanwhile prepare dressing. In a mixing bowl stir together olive oil, lemon juice, red wine vinegar, parsley, cilantro, garlic and salt. Chill while you prep the remaining salad ingredients or up to 1 day.
- In large bowl toss together quinoa, pepper, cucumber, tomato, carrot, onion and chick peas with the dressing. Serve within about 4 hours for best results. Keep salad chilled.

Nutritional Facts: 200 kcal; 30gr Carbs; 6gr Protein; 8gr Fat.

35.   GRILLED VEGGIE

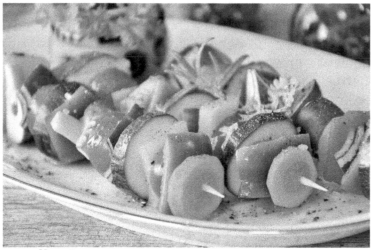

Ingredients

- 3 red bell peppers, seeded and halved
- 3 yellow squash (about 1 pound total), sliced lengthwise into 1/2-inch-thick rectangles
- 3 zucchini (about 12 ounces total), sliced lengthwise into 1/2-inch-thick rectangles
- 3 Japanese eggplant (12 ounces total), sliced lengthwise into 1/2-inch-thick rectangles
- 12 cremini mushrooms
- 1 bunch (1-pound) asparagus, trimmed
- 12 green onions, roots cut off
- 1/4 cup plus 2 tablespoons olive oil
- Salt and freshly ground black pepper
- 3 tablespoons balsamic vinegar
- 2 garlic cloves, minced
- 1 teaspoon chopped fresh Italian parsley leaves
- 1 teaspoon chopped fresh basil leaves
- 1/2 teaspoon finely chopped fresh rosemary leaves

Directions

- Place a grill pan over medium-high heat or prepare the barbecue (medium-high heat). Brush the vegetables with 1/4 cup of the oil to coat lightly. Sprinkle the vegetables with salt and pepper. Working in batches, grill the vegetables until tender and lightly charred all over, about 8 to 10 minutes for the bell peppers; 7 minutes for the yellow squash, zucchini, eggplant, and mushrooms; 4 minutes for the asparagus and green onions. Arrange the vegetables on a platter. The key to getting those great grill marks is to not shift the vegetables too frequently once they've been placed on the hot grill.
- Meanwhile, whisk the remaining 2 tablespoons of oil, balsamic vinegar, garlic, parsley, basil, and rosemary in a small bowl to blend. Add salt and pepper to taste. Drizzle the herb mixture over the vegetables. Serve the vegetables, warm or at room temperature.

Nutritional Facts: 450 kcal; 50gr Carbs; 15gr Protein; 20gr Fat.

36.   WILD RICE AND CAVOLO NERO SALAD

Ingredients
- 160 g wild rice
- 2 bunches cavolo nero, stemmed and torn into 2.5-cm pieces
- 4 tablespoons extra-virgin olive oil
- 1 teaspoon sea salt
- ¼ teaspoon freshly ground black pepper
- 6 large Brussels sprouts, trimmed and shredded
- 1 large carrot, scrubbed and shredded
- ½ red onion, finely chopped
- 2 tablespoons fresh lemon juice
- 10 g toasted pumpkin seeds

Directions
- Put the wild rice in a bowl, cover with 1 litre filtered water and leave to soak overnight at room temperature. Drain and rinse well.
- Place the rice in a small saucepan and add 625 ml filtered water. Cover, bring to the boil over a high heat, then simmer until the rice is tender and has absorbed all the liquid, about 20 minutes. Spread out the rice in a shallow baking dish and allow to cool to room temperature.
- Place the cavolo nero in a large bowl, drizzle with the olive oil, then sprinkle with the salt and pepper. Using your fingers, gently massage the leaves until wilted.
- Add the wild rice plus all the remaining ingredients and toss. Serve.

Nutritional Facts: 45 kcal; 4gr Carbs; 4gr Protein; 1gr Fat.

37.   AVOCADO, CELERY AND CITRUS SALAD

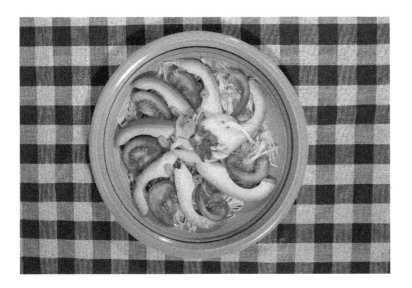

Ingredients
- 3 tablespoons Homemade Mayonnaise
- 1 tablespoon fresh lemon juice
- 1 tablespoon poppy seeds
- ½ teaspoon sea salt
- 2 blood oranges or Valencia oranges
- 1 small head romaine lettuce, torn into bite-sized pieces
- 2 avocados, stoned, peeled and each half cut into 4 slices
- 4 celery sticks, thinly sliced

Directions
1. To make the dressing, put the mayonnaise in a small bowl with the lemon juice, poppy seeds and salt and whisk together. If desired, add 1 to 2 tablespoons filtered water to thin the dressing.

2. Cut the top and bottom off an orange. Stand it on a chopping board and, using a sharp knife, cut away the rind and white pith in strips from top to bottom, following the contour of the fruit. Cut the flesh into thin rounds. Repeat with the remaining orange.
3. Divide the lettuce between 4 plates, then top equally with the orange rounds, avocado slices and celery. Drizzle some dressing over each salad and serve.

Nutritional Facts: 380 kcal; 25gr Carbs; 10gr Protein; 25gr Fat.

38. QUINOA AND BLACK BEAN SALAD WITH MEXICAN FLAVORS

Ingredients
- 170 g quinoa, rinsed and drained
- 1 x 400-g can black beans, rinsed and drained
- 2 avocados, stoned, peeled and cut into small chunks
- 1 large sweet red pepper, seeded and finely diced
- 1 large tomato, finely diced
- ½ bunch coriander, roughly chopped
- 4 tablespoons extra-virgin olive oil
- 2 tablespoons fresh lime juice
- 2 teaspoons ground cumin generous pinch of chipotle powder
- 1 teaspoon sea salt, plus more as needed

Directions
- Place the quinoa in a saucepan and cover with 500 ml filtered water. Bring to the boil over a high heat, then cover and simmer until the quinoa is almost tender and has absorbed all the liquid, about 15 minutes. Set aside, covered, for 5 minutes. Using a fork, fluff the quinoa, then spread it out in a shallow baking dish and allow to cool to room temperature.
- Transfer the cooled quinoa to a large bowl and add all the remaining ingredients. Toss until well combined, then taste and adjust the seasoning with more salt, if needed. Serve.

Nutritional Facts: 150 kcal; 20gr Carbs; 5gr Protein; 5gr Fat.

39.   WATERMELON GARBANZO & CUCUMBER SALAD

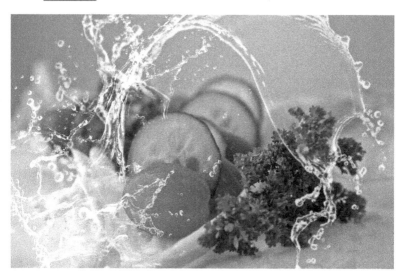

Ingredients

Dressing
- ¼ cup good olive oil
- 11/2 tablespoons balsamic vinegar
- ½ teaspoon Dijon mustard
- 1 clove garlic
- ½ teaspoon sea salt
- ½ teaspoon freshly ground black pepper

Salad
- 2 cups chopped watermelon
- 1 canned low-salt chickpeas, drained and rinsed
- ¼ small red onion, slivered and rinsed
- one box pre-washed mixed greens
- ¼ cup roughly chopped feta, French is best
- ¼ cup loosely packed, roughly torn parsley leaves

Instructions

- Chop garlic very finely. Sprinkle half of salt over garlic and mash salt and garlic together with the side of your knife, making it into a paste. Add garlic, Dijon, balsamic, salt and pepper to a bowl and whisk to combine. Slowly drizzle in olive oil, whisking constantly.
- In a large bowl, add salad ingredients and toss to combine. Drizzle dressing over greens, season with salt and pepper and serve immediately.

Nutritional Facts: 115 kcal; 7gr Carbs; 3gr Protein; 7gr Fat.

40. VEGAN GNOCCHI WITH SPINACH

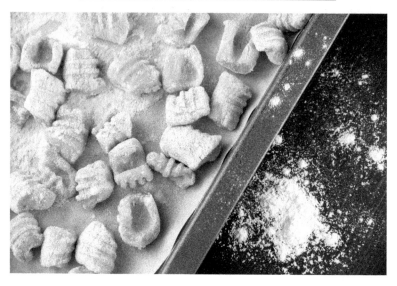

Ingredients
- 1 (16-oz.) pkg. whole-wheat potato gnocchi
- 1 (5-oz.) pkg. baby spinach
- 1 1/2 ounces Manchego cheese, grated (about 6 Tbsp.) and divided
- 3 tablespoons olive oil, divided
- 1/2 cup jarred roasted red peppers, chopped
- 1/4 cup smoked almonds
- 1 plum tomato, chopped
- 1 baguette slice, torn (about 1/2 oz.)
- 2 tablespoons sherry vinegar
- 1 garlic clove
- 1/2 teaspoon paprika
- 1/4 teaspoon crushed red pepper

Directions

- Cook gnocchi according to package directions, omitting salt and fat. Drain gnocchi; return to pan. Add spinach, 1/4 cup cheese, and 1 tablespoon olive oil; cover and let stand until spinach wilts, 2 to 3 minutes. Gently toss to combine.
- Pulse red peppers, almonds, tomato, baguette, vinegar, garlic, paprika, crushed red pepper, and remaining 2 tablespoons olive oil in a food processor until smooth, about 1 minute.
- Divide gnocchi mixture among 5 bowls. Top evenly with sauce and remaining 2 tablespoons cheese.

Nutritional Facts: 350 kcal; 70gr Carbs; 10gr Protein; 2gr Fat.

41.   CREAMY TOMATO-BASIL SOUP

Ingredients

- ½ cup (70 g) raw cashews
- 3 cups (300 g) chopped cauliflower
- 1 tablespoon (15 ml) avocado oil
- ½ cup (80 g) chopped onion
- 3 garlic cloves, minced
- 1 carrot, chopped
- 1 (32-ounce, or 908 g) jar diced tomatoes, undrained
- 2¼ to 3 cups (540 to 720 ml) water, divided
- 1 tablespoon (6 g) vegetable bouillon
- ½ cup (20 g) chopped fresh basil
- ¼ teaspoon red pepper flakes, plus more for seasoning
- Sea salt and black pepper to taste

Directions

- Soak the cashews in water and cover overnight. When ready to use, drain and rinse the cashews. If there isn't enough time to soak them overnight, soak them in boiling water for 1 hour.
- Place a steamer basket in a large pot and add 1 inch (2.5 cm) of water to the pot. Place the pot over medium-high heat. Place the cauliflower in the basket, cover, and steam for about 15 minutes until very soft. Drain.
- In a large soup pot over medium heat, heat the oil. Add the onion, garlic, and carrot. Sauté for about 10 minutes until the vegetables are softened. Stir in the tomatoes and their juices, 1½ cups (360 ml) of the water, and the vegetable bouillon. Simmer for 5 to 10 minutes.
- In a blender, combine the steamed cauliflower, drained cashews, and ¾ cup (180 ml) of water. Process for 2 to 3 minutes, or until very smooth and creamy. Remove and reserve ⅓ cup (80 ml) of cashew cream for swirling, if desired.

- Add the tomato mixture to the cashew cream in the blender. Process until smooth and creamy. Add the basil and red pepper flakes and pulse until the basil is broken up. Return the soup to the pot and rewarm.
- Taste and season with salt, black pepper, and red pepper flakes to taste. Thin with the remaining ¾ cup (180 ml) water if necessary. Serve the soup with a swirl of the reserved cashew cream, if desired.

Nutritional Facts: 180 kcal; 20gr Carbs; 5gr Protein; 10gr Fat.

42. MEXICAN QUINOA SALAD WITH GRILLED VEGETABLES

Ingredients

FOR SALSA VINAIGRETTE:

- ¾ cup (195 g) salsa
- 6 tablespoons (90 ml) red wine vinegar
- ¼ cup (60 ml) olive oil
- 1 teaspoon ground cumin
- ½ teaspoon sea salt, or to taste

FOR QUINOA SALAD:

- ½ cup (92 g) raw quinoa, cooked according to package directions
- 1 (15-ounce, or 425 g) can black beans, rinsed and drained
- 2 bell peppers, any color, cut into 1-inch (2.5 cm) squares
- 1 zucchini, cut into thick slices
- 1 cup (149 g) cherry tomatoes
- 1 tablespoon (15 ml) olive oil, plus more for the corn
- Sea salt and black pepper to taste
- 1 ear corn, husked and silks removed
- ½ cup (8 g) chopped fresh cilantro

Directions

- To make the salsa vinaigrette: In a blender, combine all the vinaigrette ingredients and pulse a few times to mix well and smooth out some of the chunkiness from the salsa. Set aside.
- To make the quinoa salad: In a large salad bowl, stir together the cooked quinoa and black beans.
- In a medium bowl, combine the bell peppers, zucchini, and tomatoes and drizzle with the oil. Season with salt and pepper to taste.
- Spray or brush the corn with oil.
- Heat an outdoor grill to medium-high heat, or heat a grill pan over medium-high heat. Add the vegetables

and cook for 3 to 5 minutes per side, long enough to have soft grill marks, being careful not to burn them.
- Cut the corn kernels from the cob and add them to the quinoa and black beans. Add the remaining grilled vegetables and mix well to combine.
- Add the cilantro and the salsa vinaigrette to the salad bowl and toss to combine and coat.

Nutritional Facts: 140 kcal; 30gr Carbs; 10gr Protein; 2gr Fat.

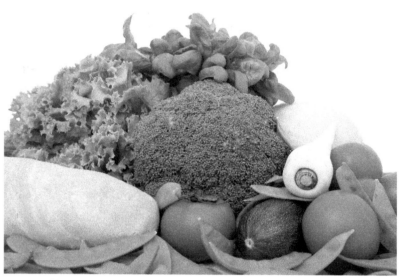

Ingredients

FOR CREAMY TAHINI DRESSING:

- ¼ cup (60 g) tahini
- ¼ cup (60 ml) olive oil
- ¼ cup (60 ml) fresh lemon juice
- ¼ cup (60 ml) white wine vinegar
- 1 tablespoon (20 g) maple syrup
- 2 teaspoons Dijon mustard
- ¼ teaspoon sea salt
- Black pepper to taste

FOR BROCCOLI SALAD:

- 8 cups (568 g) chopped broccoli
- 1 pound (454 g) bacon, cooked until crisp, drained
- 1 yellow bell pepper, seeded and chopped
- ½ cup (80 g) finely chopped red onion
- ½ cup (70 g) roasted cashews

Directions

- To make the creamy tahini dressing: In a jar or blender, combine all the dressing ingredients. Cover the jar and shake or process to combine into a creamy dressing. I prefer to use a blender because it adds air to the dressing and makes it light and ultra-creamy.
- To make the broccoli salad: Place the broccoli in a large bowl and drizzle it with the tahini dressing. Toss to coat. Refrigerate the broccoli, letting the dressing soak in, while preparing the toppings.
- When ready to serve, top the salad with the bacon, yellow bell pepper, red onion, and cashews. Toss the salad to combine and coat.
- For the best texture, refrigerate leftovers in an airtight container without the bacon and cashews, which will get soggy when stored overnight. If I know my family will not finish the whole salad at one meal, I toss the salad with the bell pepper and onion and pack half away. Refrigerate half the cooked bacon and store half the cashews separately to top the remaining salad the next day-

Nutritional Facts: 180 kcal; 15gr Carbs; 15gr Protein; 10gr Fat.

Chapter 6 : 7 Special Dessert Recipes

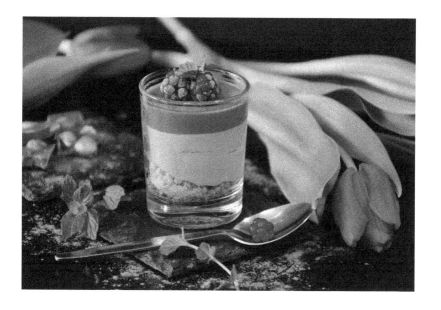

44. DARK CHOCOLATE-RASPBERRY SHORTBREAD BARS

Ingredients
FOR SHORTBREAD:
- 6 tablespoons (¾ stick; 84 g) pastured butter, at room temperature
- ¼ cup (80 g) honey
- ½ teaspoon vanilla extract
- 2 cups (193 g) blanched almond flour
- Pinch sea salt

FOR CHOCOLATE-DATE LAYER:
1. 20 ounces (560 g) pitted Medjool dates
2. ¼ cup (22 g) cacao powder
3. 3 tablespoons (42 g) pastured butter, at room temperature
4. Pinch sea salt

FOR TOPPING:
- 1 cup (125 g) fresh raspberries
- 1¾ ounces (50 g) 85% or 100% dark chocolate, melted

Directions
1. To make the shortbread: Preheat the oven to 350°F (180°C, or gas mark 4). Line an 8 × 8-inch (20 × 20 cm) baking pan with parchment paper.
2. In the bowl of a stand mixer fitted with the paddle attachment, or in a large bowl and using a hand mixer, beat the butter, honey, and vanilla on medium speed until light and fluffy.
3. Add the almond flour and salt (up to ¼ teaspoon if the butter is unsalted) and mix until there is no dry flour left.
4. Press the shortbread dough into the prepared pan. Use a pastry roller, or your hands, to flatten the dough into

a smooth and even layer. Use a fork or a chopstick to poke holes across the shortbread to ensure the dough cooks in the center as well as around the edges.

5. Bake the shortbread for 22 to 24 minutes until the top is a light golden brown. Remove from the oven and let cool fully before topping with the chocolate-date layer.
6. To make the chocolate-date layer: Place the dates in a medium-size bowl and cover them with boiling water. Let soak for about 5 minutes. Drain all the water from the dates and transfer to a food processor.
7. Add the cacao powder, butter, and salt. Process for 3 to 4 minutes, stopping to scrape the mixture from the sides about every minute or so. The mixture is ready when there are no pieces of date visible and the mixture is smooth and caramel-like. If necessary, add 1 to 2 tablespoons (15 to 30 ml) of hot water to reach the desired texture.
8. Once the shortbread has fully cooled, spread the chocolate-date mixture over the top and use wet hands to flatten it into a smooth layer.
9. To make the topping: Top the date layer with the raspberries and drizzle with the melted dark chocolate. Chill thoroughly before cutting and serving.
10. Refrigerate leftovers tightly wrapped, or in an airtight container, for up to 4 days.

Nutritional Facts: 170 kcal; 30gr Carbs; 3gr Protein; 5gr Fat.

45.   MAPLE-VEGAN MACAROONS

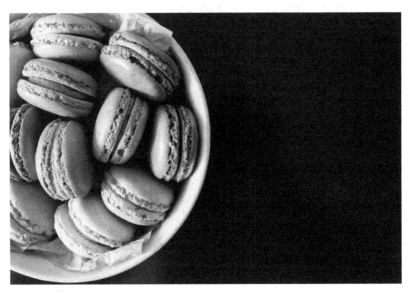

Ingredients

- ⅓ cup (107 g) maple syrup
- 1 teaspoon grass-fed gelatin
- ½ teaspoon almond exact
- ½ teaspoon vanilla extract
- 2 cups (170 g) finely shredded unsweetened coconut
- ½ cup (55 g) finely chopped pecans, plus more for garnish (optional)
- 3 ounces (85 g) unsweetened chocolate

Directions

1. Preheat the oven to 350°F (180°C, or gas mark 4). Line a baking sheet with parchment paper or a silicone baking mat.
2. In a medium-size bowl, whisk the egg whites and maple syrup until very foamy. It isn't necessary to

whisk to form peaks, like in a meringue, but the mixture should be lightened.

3. Add the gelatin, almond extract, and vanilla and whisk well.
4. Add the coconut and pecans and stir to evenly coat with the egg white mixture.
5. Use a rounded tablespoon or cookie scoop to scoop and compact the coconut batter, pressing it to hold it together well, before placing it on the prepared baking sheet. Repeat to make 20 cookies.
6. Bake the cookies for 16 to 18 minutes until lightly browned on top. Let cool fully.
7. In a double boiler, melt the unsweetened chocolate. Dip the base of each cookie into the melted chocolate to coat, placing them on a piece of wax paper to set. Use a fork to drizzle any remaining
8. chocolate on the tops of the cookies. Sprinkle the cookies with additional chopped pecans (if using).

Nutritional Facts: 200 kcal; 8gr Carbs; 3gr Protein; 15gr Fat.

46.   VANILLA-POACHED PEARS

Ingredients
1. 2 firm pears, any variety
2. 1 vanilla bean
3. 1½ cups (360 ml) water
4. 1 cup (240 ml) sweet white wine, such as Moscato
5. 1 tablespoon (20 g) maple syrup
6. 1 tablespoon (15 ml) fresh lemon juice
7. 1 cinnamon stick
8. 1 teaspoon grated lemon zest
9. ¼ cup (28 g) chopped pecans

Directions
- Halve the pears and cut out the core and seeds. Leave the stem on the pears for presentation, if desired.
- Halve the vanilla bean lengthwise so the seeds are exposed.
- In a small skillet large enough to hold the pears in a single layer, over medium heat, arrange the pears halves and add the water, white wine, maple syrup, lemon juice, vanilla bean, cinnamon stick, and lemon zest. Bring to a simmer.
- Cover the skillet and cook for 7 minutes. Remove the lid, flip the pears, and simmer for 7 minutes more to concentrate the syrup until it is reduced to about ½ cup (120 ml). If the syrup becomes too concentrated, thin it with a few tablespoons (about 45 ml) of water.
- Serve the pears with a drizzle of the white wine syrup, topped with 1 tablespoon (7 g) of chopped pecans.

Nutritional Facts: 550 kcal; 80gr Carbs; 6gr Protein; 15gr Fat.

47.   CHERRY COCONUT SORBET

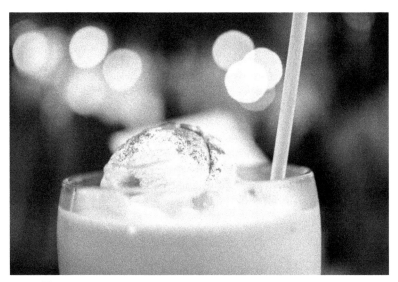

Ingredients

1. 3 cups (465 g) frozen cherries
2. ½ cup (120 ml) coconut milk

Directions

- In a high-speed blender or food processor, combine the cherries and coconut milk. Process on high speed until smooth and creamy. It helps to use a blender with a tamper stick, or to stop the food processor and scrape down the sides a few times throughout the process.
- The dessert is a soft-serve consistency and delicious served right away. If you'd like to serve this sorbet in scoops, transfer it to a shallow container, cover, and freeze for 1 to 2 hours.
- Freeze leftovers in an ice-cube tray, then store the sorbet cubes in an airtight container. Let the cubes thaw slightly for 10 to 15 minutes before putting them

into the food processor to re-blend into a creamy dessert.

Nutritional Facts: 100 kcal; 20gr Carbs; 2gr Protein; 1gr Fat.

48. SNEAKY BLACK BEAN BROWNIES

Ingredients

- 1 (15-ounce) can low-sodium black beans
- ¼ avocado
- 1 tablespoon coconut oil, melted
- 2 tablespoons nut butter (preferably cashew butter)
- 2 teaspoons pure vanilla extract
- 1/3 cup ground flaxseed
- 1 large pasture-raised egg
- 1/3 cup pure maple syrup
- 1 tablespoon granulated monk fruit sweetener, for baking (optional)
- ¼ teaspoon sea salt
- ½ teaspoon baking powder
- 1/3 cup unsweetened organic cacao powder
- ½ cup dairy-free dark chocolate chips (preferably sweetened with monk fruit or stevia)

Directions

1. Drain the beans and rinse them well, letting them dry in a sieve. Preheat the oven to 350°F. Line an 8 x 8-inch baking dish with parchment paper.
2. Place the avocado, coconut oil, nut butter, vanilla extract, and beans in a food processor. Blend for 30 seconds until combined. Scrape the sides if needed.
3. Add the ground flaxseed, egg, maple syrup, monk fruit (if using), salt, and baking powder and process for 20 seconds.
4. Sift the cacao powder into the food processor bowl and process for 10 seconds. Scrape the sides and process for another 5 seconds. The batter should be thick and sticky.
5. Spread half of the mixture in the baking dish, sprinkle on the chocolate chips, and spread the rest of the

batter on top. Smooth evenly with a spatula or the back of a spoon.

6. Place the baking dish on the top rack of the oven and bake for 25 minutes, or until the center of the brownie in the pan no longer jiggles. If testing with a toothpick, the toothpick should come out a bit sticky for fudgy brownies. Remove from the oven and let cool completely before slicing into 14 pieces. Store leftovers in an airtight container in the fridge for up to 5 days.

Nutritional Facts: 60 kcal; 8gr Carbs; 2gr Protein; 20gr Fat.

49.   BANANA SWEET WITH COCONUT CREAM

Ingredients
- 5 bananas, Cut into 2-inch pieces
- 2 cups coconut milk, Low fat is fine
- 4 tablespoons granulated sugar
- 1/2 teaspoon salt
- 1 cinnamon stick

GARNISH
1. 1/4 cup toasted coconut
2. 1 mango, peeled pitted and cubed (optional)

Directions
1. In a saucepan, heat the coconut milk with the cinnamon, sugar and salt, and cook gently until the sugar has dissolved. Add the banana pieces and cook gently for 5 minutes.
2. Remove cinnamon and discard.
3. Divide the mixture into 6-8 small bowls and serve warm.

Nutritional Facts: 100 kcal; 14gr Carbs; 20gr Protein; 1gr Fat.

50.   DARK CHOCOLATE COOKIES

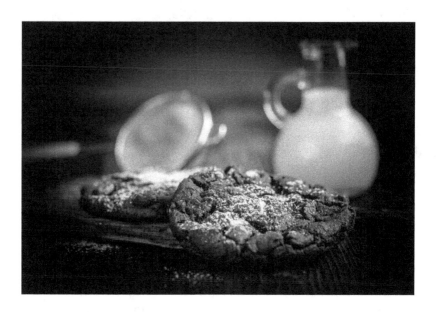

Ingredients
1. 1 cup (125g) all-purpose flour (spoon & leveled)
2. 1/3 cup (26g) natural unsweetened cocoa powder*
3. 1/3 cup (26g) Hershey's special dark cocoa powder*
4. 1 teaspoon baking soda
5. 1/8 teaspoon salt
6. 1/2 cup (115g) unsalted butter, softened to room temperature
7. 1/2 cup (100g) granulated sugar
8. 1/2 cup (100g) packed light or dark brown sugar
9. 1 large egg, at room temperature
10. 1 teaspoon pure vanilla extract
11. 2 Tablespoons (30ml) milk
12. 1 cup (180g) semi-sweet or dark chocolate chunks and/or chips, plus a few more for topping*
13. sea salt for sprinkling

Instructions

- Whisk the flour, cocoa powders, baking soda and salt together until combined. Set aside.
- In a large bowl using a hand-held or stand mixer fitted with a paddle attachment, beat the butter for 1 minute on medium speed until completely smooth and creamy. Add the granulated sugar and brown sugar and beat on medium high speed until fluffy and light in color. Beat in egg and vanilla on high speed. Scrape down the sides and bottom of the bowl as needed.
- On low speed, slowly mix the dry ingredients into the wet ingredients until combined. The cookie dough will be thick. Switch to high speed and beat in the milk, then the chocolate chips. The cookie dough will be sticky. Cover dough tightly with aluminum foil or plastic wrap and chill for at least 3 hours and up to 3 days. Chilling is mandatory for this cookie dough. I always chill mine overnight.
- Remove cookie dough from the refrigerator and allow to sit at room temperature for 20 minutes– if the cookie dough chilled longer than 3 hours, let it sit at room temperature for about 30 minutes. This makes the cookie dough easier to scoop and roll.
- Preheat oven to 350°F (177°C). Line two large baking sheets with parchment paper or silicone baking mats. (Always recommended for cookies.) Set aside.
- Scoop and roll balls of dough, about 2 Tablespoons of dough each, into balls. Place on the baking sheets and sprinkle with a little sea salt.
- Bake the cookies for 10 minutes. My oven has hot spots and yours may too- so be sure to rotate the pan once during bake time. The baked cookies will look extremely soft in the centers when you remove them from the oven. Allow to cool for 5 minutes on the cookie sheet. During this time, you can press a few more chocolate chips/chunks into the top of the warm cookies– this is just for looks. You can also sprinkle with a little more sea salt as well. The cookies will

slightly deflate as you let them cool. Transfer to cooling rack to cool completely.

Nutritional Facts: 600 kcal; 30gr Carbs; 8gr Protein; 40gr Fat.

CPSIA information can be obtained
at www.ICGtesting.com
Printed in the USA
LVHW052020210621
690769LV00012B/1857